YOU– AFTER CHILDBIRTH

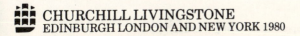

KW-249-929

EXERCISES AND ADVICE FOR THE NEW MOTHER

JULIE McKENNA, M.C.S.P.,
Senior Obstetric Physiotherapist,
Royal Free Hospital, London

MARGARET POLDEN, M.C.S.P.,
Senior Obstetric Physiotherapist,
Royal Free Hospital and Hammersmith Hospital
Teacher, National Childbirth Trust

MARGARET WILLIAMS, M.C.S.P., M.A.O.T.,
Senior Obstetric Physiotherapist,
Victoria Hospital, Barnet
Advanced Teacher, National Childbirth Trust

Foreword by
Josephine Barnes,
D.B.E., M.A., D.M., F.R.C.P., F.R.C.S.,
F.R.C.O.G.(Hon.) F.R.C.P.(Ireland)
President, Association of Chartered Physiotherapists
in Obstetrics and Gynaecology

CHURCHILL LIVINGSTONE
EDINBURGH LONDON AND NEW YORK 1980

CHURCHILL LIVINGSTONE
Medical Division of Longman Group Limited

Distributed in the United States of America by
Churchill Livingstone Inc.,
19 West 44th Street, New York, N.Y. 10036,
and by associated companies, branches
and representatives throughout the world.

First published 1980

ISBN 0 443 02128 7

British Library Cataloguing in Publication Data
McKenna, Julie
  You, after childbirth.
  1. Physical fitness for women
  2. Postnatal care
  I. Title II. Polden, Margaret
  III. Williams, Margaret, *Lady, b. 1915*
  613.7'045   GV439   79–41249

Printed by Singapore Offset Printing (Pte) Ltd.

FOREWORD

I am delighted to welcome this booklet on postnatal rehabilitation and to write the foreword for it.

Antenatal care has changed and advanced remarkably in this century, but this may often appear to be at the expense of postnatal care. The days and weeks which follow childbirth are vital for the future health of the mother and thus for the well-being of her child and the future of the family unit. Nowadays, with smaller families, many young mothers are isolated and lack the help and support they received in former days. Many leave hospital after a day or two and are flung into an exhausting and exacting routine of caring for the baby and the household—with little time or energy to care for themselves.

It is right therefore that everything should be done to ensure that the mother not only regains her figure but also keeps herself in a state of physical and thus of mental fitness for the tasks which face her.

I hope this booklet will be made widely available in maternity units, where nowadays the majority of babies are born, so that all mothers can have the benefit of the excellent advice it contains.

London, 1980   Josephine Barnes

PREFACE

You – After Childbirth replaces *Your Baby and Your Figure*, a booklet of both antenatal and postnatal exercises, first written for the Obstetric Association of Chartered Physiotherapists in 1961 and revised several times since then.

The present booklet, again commissioned by the Society (now re-named the Association of Chartered Physiotherapists in Obstetrics and Gynaecology) is rather more than a revision. The authors have concentrated entirely on the postnatal period in order to

YOU-AFTER CHILDBIRTH

provide comprehensive advice to the new mother.

We should like to thank Dame Josephine Barnes, President of the Association of Chartered Physiotherapists in Obstetrics and Gynaecology, for her help and encouragement and for writing the foreword. We are also grateful to the Royal College of Midwives, the Health Visitors Association and other doctors, midwives, health visitors and physiotherapists as well as young parents, for their helpful criticism and comments.

London, 1980
J.M.
M.P.
M.W.

CONTENTS

CAESAREAN SECTION

MORE POSTNATAL EXERCISES

YOUR BABY

Immediately after your child is born you may feel a tremendous surge of love or a slight feeling of detachment towards this new baby, which may not look quite so beautiful as you had expected. Do not worry or feel guilty if the latter emotion is uppermost. Falling in love with a baby is like any other love affair: sometimes it is instantaneous; sometimes it takes a long time to develop.

You will probably go to one of the postnatal wards about one hour after your baby is born. You may still be elated, hungry, talkative and on top of the world, wanting to touch your baby and unable to take your eyes off him; or you may long just to be left in peace to go to

sleep—particularly if you have had a lot of medication.
During the next few days you will gradually get used to
the very busy routine of the maternity ward; you will pass
through the phase of feeling awkward and slowly learn to
feed and care for your baby. You will have the fun of
watching the things he can do, the noises he makes and
the expressions that pass over his face. If your baby
cannot be with you and is sent to the special care nursery,
spend as much time with him as possible. There are
many reasons why a baby may need more attention than
can be given to him in a busy ward.

YOUR BODY

A few hours after the birth you will begin to think about yourself as well as about the baby. Your body may feel that it has done a very hard day's work, as indeed it has. Your perineum (the area around the vagina and rectum; see p. 9) may give you a curious mixture of sensations: the back may be sore if you have had stitches and the front feel as if it does not belong to you, so much so that you may be unaware of any feeling of wanting to pass water. Your abdomen (tummy), may be rather flabby and not as flat as you had hoped. If you have had an epidural anaesthetic there may still be some slight numbness or weakness between your waist and your knees. You may even have a backache or headache.

Getting up

If, for some reason, you have to stay in bed, practise deep breathing and move your legs and feet frequently. However, if you had a straightforward labour you will probably be allowed up to go to the toilet, accompanied by a nurse, in about six hours and to have a bath a little later. Before getting out of bed for the first time, take one or two really deep breaths, do some up and down movements with your feet, then sit on the side of the bed and swing your legs vigorously a few times. Finally, stand up slowly, brace your abdominal muscles, try to pull up the pelvic floor muscles between your legs and bend and stretch your knees once or twice before walking slowly to the toilet. If you have any difficulty in passing water do the pelvic floor exercise on p. 11 a few times and it may help you to start. At first you will probably find that you are still walking as if you were pregnant. Correct posture becomes easier as you practise the exercises and get used to your changed shape.

A good hint for recalling the right way to stand is to lie flat on your bed with one pillow under your head; then stretch the crown of your head up towards the top of the bed and your heels down to the bottom and flatten all the curves of your spine. This will remind you of the muscles that need to be braced when you stand up.

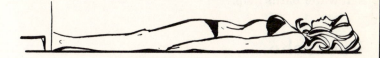

After pains

Your body will slowly begin to feel normal again. For the first few days you will have a heavy period-like discharge (lochia) and may even pass a few clots. Save the pad if you notice one of these and let the ward-sister check it. The lochia will gradually change from red to brown to a slight, whitish discharge.

You may have 'after pains', that is contractions like mild labour or period pains caused by the gradual shrinking of your uterus back to its normal size. These tend to be worse after second and subsequent babies and often start when you put the baby to your breast. The same hormone circulating in the blood stream is responsible for the contractions and the flow of milk.

Stitches

Perineal stitches can be very uncomfortable, particularly if there is also bruising of the tissues. The discomfort tends to be at its worst four to five days after delivery, but after that there is often quite a marked improvement. Frequent gentle contractions of the pelvic floor muscles help by improving the local circulation and so reducing the swelling around the stitches. You will be offered pain-relieving tablets, and, in addition, the doctor may suggest that you have some treatment to improve the circulation further; this may be a form of heat such as infra-red rays, or the application of an ice pack. Many people find that salt water baths help.

Backache

There is a normal softening and slackening of the joints of the spine and pelvis during pregnancy, and if you sit, stand or lift badly while your body is still slack, this may give rise to backache. Read, and try to put into practice the sections on exercise and everyday activities. Boards under the mattress may help, as will plenty of rest either flat on your back or on your abdomen, as on pages 18 to 19. While lying down, tighten your buttocks frequently as hard as you can as if you were trying to grip a £5 note between them.

Breasts

When you first start breast-feeding your baby, your breasts produce colostrum, a yellowish fluid which is protective and highly nourishing. This gradually changes to milk a few days after delivery. If your baby has been put to the breast regularly this may be a smooth process with no discomfort, but sometimes your breasts feel quite normal at one moment and a few hours later they are swollen, hot and aching. The first few feeds after the milk-flow starts may be a little uncomfortable. Seek advice from your midwife as to whether to put your baby to the breast more frequently or to draw off some of the milk. She will show you how to do this. A flannel soaked in ice-cold water, wrung out and applied to each breast in turn can help to relieve discomfort, whichever way you are feeding. You will also need to wear a strong, well-fitting bra night and day.

PROBLEMS

The 'blues'

Most people have heard about 'baby blues' and quite a lot of mothers do go through a period of weepiness and depression, often lasting anything from a few hours to a few days. The main cause of this is probably the rapid reversal of the hormone changes which occurred during pregnancy; the same sort of thing happens around a menstrual period. Worry about some aspect of the baby's care or an increase in your discomforts are often additional causes. Sometimes it is just tiredness or a reaction to the big effort of labour and the dawning realisation of your new responsibilities. Some women are simply homesick for their husbands, friends or children. Adequate rest can be a great help in overcoming this, not only at night but in naps during the day and by the deliberate practice of relaxation which you probably learned during antenatal classes. If your depression continues when you go home, do tell your health visitor or doctor; help is available for this very distressing condition.

Baby worries

If you are worried about the baby, do not ask one of the junior staff but talk to the midwife in charge of the ward or to the doctor. They will be able to reassure you that such conditions as jaundice are very common in new-born babies and will clear up in a few days. The paediatrician will be responsible for the baby and your obstetrician will continue to look after you. When you go home, the health visitor (whom you may have already met antenatally) will call on you to discuss your own and your baby's progress. She will tell you about the community health clinic or your own doctor's baby clinic if he holds one. If you are discharged from hospital early, your community midwife will care for you at first.

Sometimes it can be reassuring to join a local parents' group where you will soon discover that other mothers have problems similar to your own. Remember that you will be with your baby every day and you will soon develop a sort of sixth sense about what is right for him.

BACK TO NORMAL

After the birth you will gradually feel better as you start moving about and doing some exercises for your figure. Two groups of muscles need strengthening—the *pelvic floor* muscles and the *abdominal* muscles.

The pelvic floor muscles

These form a sling-like floor to the 'basin' of the pelvis and surround the exits of the vagina (birth canal) the urethra (the passage for urine from the bladder) and the anus (back passage).

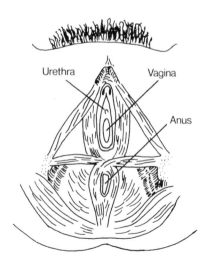

Urethra

Vagina

Anus

They have three very *vital* functions:

1. They affect the efficiency of the bladder. (You may have noticed a bladder weakness during pregnancy. This is probably due to hormone changes which affect the muscles.)
2. They support the contents of the pelvis, e.g. the bladder, bowel and uterus.
3. They affect the enjoyment of sexual intercourse for both partners.

In recent years, due to several factors, there has been a marked improvement in the condition of the pelvic floor after childbirth. Perhaps the most important of these factors, is the antenatal and postnatal teaching and exercising of the muscles. Controlling the length of the second stage of labour (many hospitals like to limit this to an hour or less) is also beneficial. Lastly the use of episiotomy (a small cut made during delivery to increase the outlet of the vagina where the alternative might be a bad tear or over-stretching) and the careful stitching of any tears or episiotomy, has helped to minimise the trauma to this area.

The abdominal muscles

These consist of layers of muscle fibres, some of them passing straight up and down the abdomen, some across and some in an oblique direction. The vertical fibres, called the rectus abdominis muscle (see diagram p. 11), form a double band which tends to separate during pregnancy. Together, these groups form a natural 'corset' supporting the abdominal organs and also the spine, and weakness of this 'corset' after childbirth is a common cause of backache.

During pregnancy your abdominal muscles obviously became very stretched. Your posture was altered and you

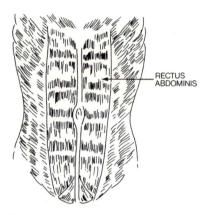

RECTUS ABDOMINIS

probably noticed an increase in the natural hollow of your back. This will gradually correct itself during the postnatal period as the abdominal muscles are strengthened. It is not necessary to do long lists of exercises—and this would not be practical for the busy young mother. There may be an obstetric physiotherapist to guide you but, if not, the following exercises, if practised carefully, will start to build up the strength of the muscles of the abdomen and pelvic floor. If you wish to do more later, there is a longer list at the end of this booklet.

Exercises

Pelvic floor muscles
1. Perhaps you have already practised this exercise in your ante-natal classes. Even if you have had stitches and are feeling sore, it is still a good idea to try and practise it gently as soon as possible. Some of the discomfort will be due to swelling and this can be relieved by contracting and relaxing the muscles.

Close up the ring of muscle around the back passage (as if you are stopping a motion)—now try to tighten the birth canal in the same way (as if you were trying to stop yourself passing water). Hold both muscles tight for as long as you can.

Try to do this important exercise regularly during the day—aim at holding the muscle tense while you count slowly to four (i.e. four seconds).

Do this four times after each visit to the toilet. This guarantees frequent practice and you will soon feel the muscles getting stronger. (Check the improvement periodically by trying to stop the flow of urine in mid-stream.)

Luckily, most of us are vain and determined to get back a good figure after having a baby. *But always remember that strong pelvic floor muscles are just as important as strong abdominal muscles.*

Abdominal muscles

2. Lie on your back with your knees bent. Put one hand under the small of your back. Flatten your back down onto your hand and at the same time tilt your pelvis towards your face. Hold it—relax. This is to strengthen the double band of muscle fibres which pass down the middle of the abdomen and to pull them together.

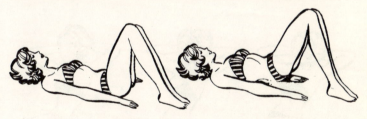

3. Lie on your back with one knee bent and one knee straight. Rest one hand lightly on your abdomen just above the straight leg. Lengthen the straight leg by stretching down with the heel. Now slide the heel up towards you *keeping the knee straight* and shortening the leg at the waist. As you do this *tighten the muscle under your hand*. Do this a few times and then change legs and repeat. (This is for the muscle fibres responsible for the side-bending movements.)

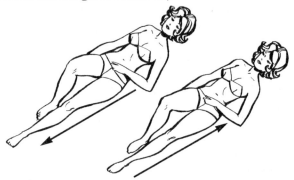

4. Lie on your back with both knees bent. Flatten your back down onto the bed or floor (thus tightening the abdominal muscles). Keeping this position, roll both knees together over to one side as far as possible. Now bring them upright and relax the abdomen. Repeat the whole series of movements to the other side. (This is for the muscle fibres which perform the twisting movements of the trunk.)

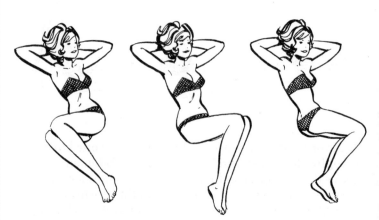

Some mothers will be ready to start exercises within hours of delivery, while for others, rest at that early time will be far more important than exercise. See how *you* feel but do remember that many of your discomforts will be relieved by activity. This applies particularly to the perineal area if it has been stitched. Try to start the pelvic floor routine as early as possible and this will begin to relieve the discomfort. A guide-line for the abdominal exercises is to start by doing each one five times twice daily and increase by one a day until twenty and keep at this number.

If you notice that your tummy bulges as you are exercising and you are unable to keep the muscles braced, you are progressing too quickly. Concentrate on Exercise 2 until this improves. Always remember that general tiredness can be due to weakness of muscles, so aim to strengthen them as soon as possible. It is usually better to do exercises on a mat or blanket on the floor, but you may have to do them on your bed while in hospital.

As your muscles get stronger you will find it easier to stand and walk with a good posture (see page 17).

COPING WITH DAILY LIVING

In hospital

You may need to feed your baby six to eight times a day or more at first. If you make sure that you are really comfortable when you do this, you will be able to look forward to each feed and use it as a chance to rest and relax. If you are uncomfortable and tense, whether you are breast- or bottle-feeding, the baby will sense it and he will not feed so well. You can relax your hunched shoulders by pulling them down (so making your neck longer) and then releasing the pull.

Because your stitches will be sore, it may be necessary to relieve the pressure on this area, by sitting on a pillow

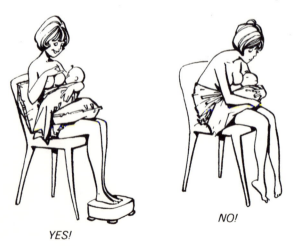

YES!

NO!

or an air-ring. Otherwise, make sure that you put your bottom right to the back of the chair. Have a pillow behind your waist and one or two on your lap to raise the baby and avoid sagging forward.

When you stand up, bend forward from your hips, brace your abdomen, and push off with your hands. Bracing your abdomen, will also help when lowering yourself down into a chair.

If you feed your baby in bed, have the backrest up behind your back so that you are well supported.

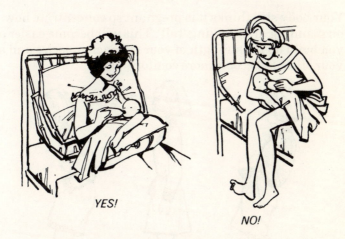

YES!

NO!

It may be possible to feed your baby lying on your side.

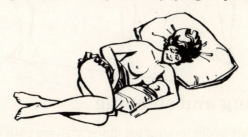

Many women find that in the beginning they seem to have no energy and very little time for exercises. It is a good idea to get used to pulling in the abdominal muscles and lifting the pelvic floor muscles whilst the baby is feeding—it will not bother him at all. If you could manage to do these exercises just a few times at each feed it would add up to quite a bit in a day.

Standing and walking

Your body still thinks it is pregnant so concentrate now on standing and walking 'tall'. This will become easier as you build up the strength of your stomach muscles and as your stitches become more comfortable.

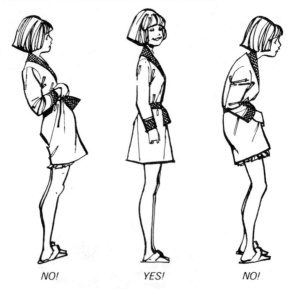

NO!　　　　YES!　　　　NO!

Resting and sleeping

If possible avoid having too many visitors both in hospital and when you first get home. A good rest on your own is often preferable. Choose from the following positions:

1. On your back (with a pillow under your thighs).
2. On your side (arranging the pillow to take the pressure off your breasts).
3. Face downwards (with one pillow under your waist and one under your head and shoulders).

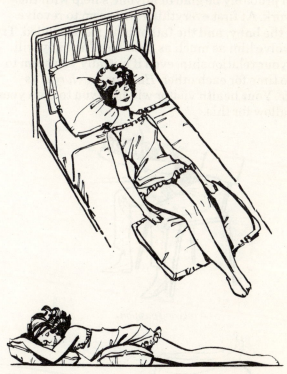

The last position is particularly comfortable for sore bottoms or aching backs.

To get up—bend your knees up high, roll onto your side and push yourself up with your hands. Remember: *all movement is made easier if the abdomen is held tense.*

At home

Because of your new responsibilities you will be wise to resume normal life gradually. If you can arrange to have someone with you at home for the first week or so, you will be able to devote all your time and energy to the baby. Perhaps the best person is the baby's father; but you will probably be glad of anyone's help with the housework. At first everything will seem to revolve around the baby, and the father may feel excluded. Try and involve him as much as possible. The baby will enrich your relationship, even if initially you seem to have no time for each other. *Have as much rest as possible.* Your health visitor will help you to plan your day to allow for this.

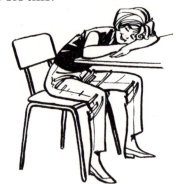

A relaxing position

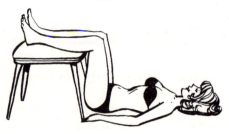

A relaxing position

When bending to pick up anything from the floor, keep your back straight and bend your knees. If you need to lift anything heavy, brace your pelvic floor muscles as well.

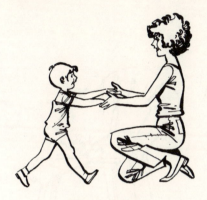

Brace pelvic floor

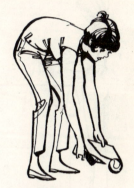

*Try not to stoop
with a rounded back
when doing the housework*

Try to choose a pram that is the correct height for you.

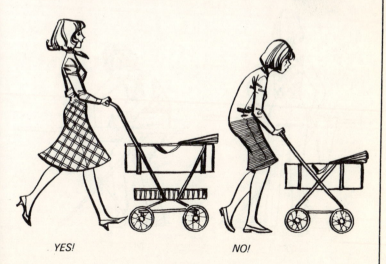

YES!   *NO!*

If you are going to have a worktop for changing your baby, be sure to arrange things so that you do not have to bend over.

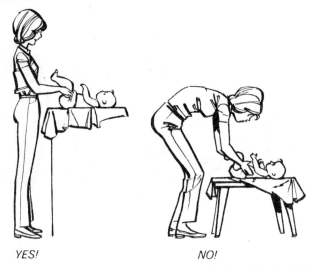

YES!   NO!

Try to have all work surfaces around the right height.

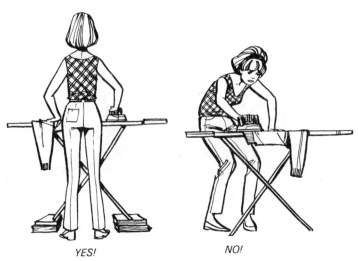

YES!   NO!

A carrying sling will be most useful if you want to take the baby shopping or if he cries a great deal. The type that is worn on your chest at first and later on your back is better than the sling which goes across your body because it leaves both your arms free.

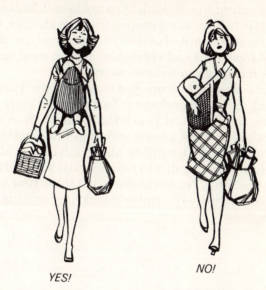

YES!   NO!

Diet

During your pregnancy you will probably have gained between one and two stone in weight. Apart from the weight of the baby, placenta, uterus etc., between 10 and 12 lb will be stored as fat in various parts of your body. This fat will be broken down and used in the production of breast milk. Many women find that breast-feeding makes them lose weight very quickly so that they soon have their pre-pregnancy figure again. However, some women find that breast-feeding makes them very hungry indeed, and these women will lose their excess weight later.

In the same way that you were careful to have a well-balanced diet during pregnancy, so it is important to continue eating wisely whilst you are breast feeding. A good rule is to have some protein (fish, meat, eggs, cheese, milk) a small amount of carbohydrate (bread, potatoes etc.) and fresh fruit and vegetables at each meal, and to drink as much as you feel necessary.

If your milk supply drops you may be advised to eat and drink more and perhaps to feed the baby more often. If you are worried about your weight, cut down on fried foods, cakes, biscuits, sweets and chocolates, potatoes and bread. Your doctor will be able to advise you about a safe weight-reducing diet to follow whilst you continue feeding the baby. Try not to worry if it takes time to regain your figure—remember it took nine months to grow the baby!

Sex

Some doctors advise waiting at least two weeks after the birth of the baby before making love.
Others say that as soon as you feel like it you can go ahead. If in doubt, seek the advice of your own doctor. It may be some time before you feel comfortable enough, depending partly on how quickly your stitches heal. However, many people lose their normal desire for a time. You can show love for each other in many ways before you attempt full intercourse. K-Y jelly has helped many people over postnatal vaginal dryness; it can be bought from any chemist. Remember that breast feeding is not a foolproof contraceptive, so be sure to consult your G.P. or family planning clinic if this matter has not been discussed with you in the hospital.

CAESAREAN SECTION

About 10 to 12 per cent of women will need a caesarean section to make sure that their baby will be normal and healthy after it is born.

For whatever reason this operation is considered necessary, do remember that it does not mean that you have failed in any way by not pushing the baby out yourself. Instead, you should try and accept that, thanks to modern skills and techniques, both you and your baby have been brought safely through a situation that could have resulted in damage. Next time you may be able to have a normal delivery.

When you wake after the anaesthetic you will feel very tired and 'woozy'. Your stomach will be extremely sore and you will probably have a drip in your arm, and perhaps a small tube (catheter) in your urethra (front passage) to keep the bladder empty. Usually, the incision will have been made low down across your abdomen so that it will easily be covered by a bikini afterwards. Sometimes, though, the doctor will have made a vertical incision. In both these cases, the stitches will be covered by a soft dressing.

Advice for the first few days

1. It is important to rid your lungs of any remaining anaesthetic, so take frequent deep breaths moving your ribs sideways and stressing the breath out. You may find that you need to cough some mucus from your chest; it is less painful if you support your abdomen with your hands while you do this, and make your cough more of a short sharp pant, rather than a throaty noise which will be much more uncomfortable. If you do not cough the phlegm up you will delay your recovery.

2. It is essential for your circulation to move your feet and legs after an operation. The following are the exercises you should do often until you are able to move more freely and comfortably:

a. Bend and stretch your ankles vigorously several times.
b. Circle your feet round and round.
c. Press your knees hard on the bed and tighten your buttocks at the same time.
d. Bend alternate legs keeping your heels on the bed.
e. Practise the deep breathing already mentioned—it will also aid your circulation.

3. You will, of course, have help getting out of bed at first. Some hospitals have beds which can be raised or lowered, otherwise use a stool to step down and up. Any movement will be made less painful by bracing your abdomen first. Shift yourself to the side of the bed gradually, lifting your bottom over by pressing your fists down hard. Then using your hands if necessary, take one leg and then the other over the edge so that you can slip forward and stand. Try and keep yourself as straight as possible. Then walk slowly to a chair, holding your stomach with your hands at first. It is easier to sit on a high firm chair that has arms which you can grasp as you bend your knees and lower your weight well back on to the chair seat. Sometimes, the soreness, abdominal wind and 'after pains' (see p. 4) will be so bad that you will find yourself becoming very tense. This is when you can use your antenatal relaxation technique plus the slow, deep breathing.

4. If you do have a problem with your chest, it is important to sit upright; call the nurses if you slip down so that they can help you up again. You may find that your back begins to ache with the constant sitting up. As soon as your chest is clear it will be more comfortable to ease yourself down the bed to lie on your side with your abdomen and legs supported by pillows.

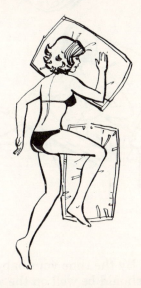

5. Feeding your baby will need a little practice. It might be uncomfortable to cuddle him to you in the crook of your arm because there will be pressure on your abdomen. Instead, try tucking him under your arm so that his legs and body are by your side, and his face towards the breast. One mother found that the bed table made a comfortable support (see illustrations p.27).

After a couple of days, you can begin to pull your abdominal muscles in gently and then gradually add the normal postnatal exercises as advised by your

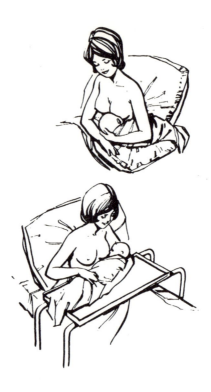

physiotherapist. By the time your baby is 8 to 10 weeks old, your figure should be well on the way back to normal. Do not worry, though, if it takes a little longer than it does for the mothers who had a vaginal delivery.

MORE POST-NATAL EXERCISES

To flatten the abdomen and slim the hips

1. Lie on your back with both knees bent. Pull in your abdominal muscles and, keeping them firmly braced, lift your head and shoulders and stretch your hands towards your feet. You can lift higher each day until you actually sit up and then lower back slowly.

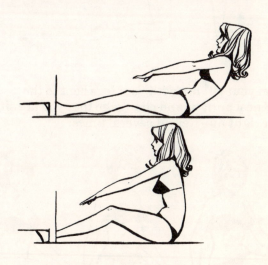

2. Kneel on all fours. Pull your abdominal muscles in and bend your right knee up to your chin; then stretch it out behind you before putting it down. Repeat with the left leg.

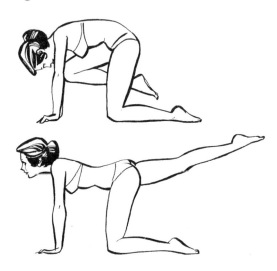

3. Sit on your left hip with your legs bent to the right. Kneel upright and change so that you are sitting on your right hip. Repeat several times.

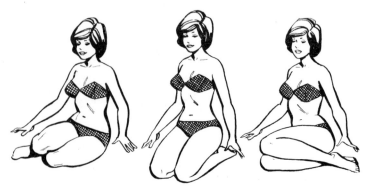

4. Lie on your back with both knees bent up high and your toes tucked under something heavy. Tuck in your abdominal muscles and stretch your right hand across your chest and reach down towards your left ankle. Rest back again and relax your abdomen. Repeat to the other side.

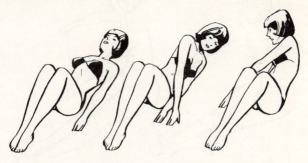

5. Lie on your back with your arms stretched out sideways. Lift your right leg and take it over towards your left hand twisting from the waist and keeping your arms flat on the floor. Put it down and repeat with your left leg.

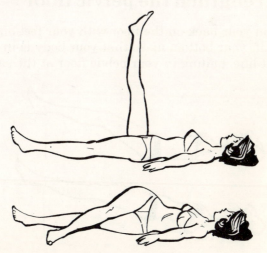

6. Sit on the floor with your back straight and your arms stretched forward. Hold your abdomen in and then 'walk' forward on your bottom, then 'walk' backwards.

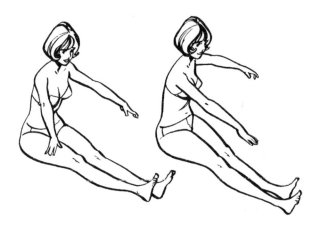

To strengthen the pelvic floor

7. Lie on your back on the floor with your feet on a stool. Lift your bottom up so that your body is in a straight line, pulling in your pelvic floor at the same time.

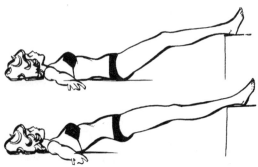

Remember that it is important to exercise these muscles often, and it can be done in many situations, for example standing at the sink, waiting in queues, etc.

To shape up the breasts

8. Sitting, standing or kneeling hold your arms horizontally in front of you with each hand gripping the opposite upper arm just above the elbow. Grip each arm tightly, and push the arms together; hold it, and then relax. You will feel your breasts being lifted by the muscles which support them, and strengthening them may help to prevent the breasts from sagging. But *more important than any exercise is a well-fitting bra.*

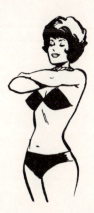

Apart from these special exercises you will soon feel well enough to take long walks with the baby and this is very good general exercise. Swimming is another sport you will be able to enjoy with the baby, and many swimming baths have special mother and baby classes.

Unless you have kept up activities such as badminton, yoga, keep fit classes or cycling during pregnancy, it is better *not* to start again until you are passed as fit after your postnatal check up. Then start gently and gradually. Remember: although pregnancy and labour are normal events, your body has been under a strain and needs time to recover. If you have no time to do anything else, at least pull in your abdomen every time you think about it and pull up your pelvic floor every time you go to the toilet.

WHAT NOT TO DO

Do not do any exercises which involve lying on your back and either lifting both legs in the air or sitting up with knees straight on the floor. Such exercises put an undue strain on your back, abdomen and pelvic floor.